I0427964

The DASH Diet

The Beginner's Guide to the DASH Diet – Includes 25 Recipes!

Table of Contents

Introduction

The DASH (Dietary Approaches to Stop Hypertension) Diet is a diet that was originally created to help lower blood pressure. However, many are now finding that this diet works even better for those that are looking to lose weight. This diet has been known to speedup weight loss and can have you looking and feeling physically younger.

In present day, dieting seems to be difficult for almost everyone. There so many people complaining of failed attempts at trying the latest fad diets. The problem with these fad-diets is that the results never last long, and the individual is always left with a growling stomach and lighter pockets. The DASH Diet is nothing like the diets that you see on TV and read in magazines. This diet produces long-lasting results that will stick with you for years to come.

Many are in the dark when it comes to weight loss and getting their health under control. It is my hope that may book, **The DASH Diet:** *The Beginner's Guide to the DASH Diet* can shed some light on how easy the road to weight loss and health really is. This diet will definitely take you in the direction that you need to make room for you to begin living a healthier and happier lifestyle.

Chapter 1 – How does the DASH Diet work?

There is a difference between dieting and a diet. Many people don't understand the ambiguity of the word diet. However, this can be easily explained. A diet can be described as the types of food that any living specimen eats on the day to day. Dieting or to diet on the other hand, means to restrict oneself to a specific amount of food and calories to achieve a desired weight.

So one thing that the DASH Diet meal plan is not about is dieting. It's all about eating for better health. The DASH Diet is a regimen that is all about eating some great tasting holistic foods and lowering sodium intake. This diet will assist you in making an easy transition into a healthy lifestyle. It's recommended for longevity, weight loss, reversing the effects of hypertension, diabetes, and more. This diet is rich in foods that contain potassium, magnesium, and calcium, which are some of the nutrients needed to keep high blood pressure at bay.

Studies have shown that the DASH Diet has resulted in more weight loss than the average low-fat, low-calorie diet. This is because this diet causes the body's metabolism to increase, which in return helps the body burn an increased amount of calories and get rid of some of the dead calories in the body.

What does this diet consist of?

You can look to enjoy high consumption of whole-grains, healthy fats, low-fat or fat-free dairy, fruits, vegetables, lean meat, fish, and poultry. You will also moderately enjoy small, fulfilling servings of sweets, pulses and legumes. Sweets and heavier red meats are fine, but eat VERY OCCASIONALLY.

Let's take a look at exactly how healthy of a serving you will be enjoying from each of the food groups mentioned above:

- Six to Eight Servings of **Grains** per day
- Four to Five Servings of **Vegetables** per day
- Four to Five Servings of **Fruit** per day
- Two to Three Servings of **Low-Fat or Non-Fat Dairy** per day
- Up to Six Servings of **Lean Meat, Poultry, or Fish** per day
- Four to Five Servings of **Nuts, Seeds, and Legumes** per week
- Two to Three Servings of **Fats and Oils** per day
- Up to Five Servings of **Sweets** per week

The intent of this diet is to lead you into the finding you finding your ideal nutritional balance, and to get you in the habit of eating more vegetables, more protein, and finding you ideal nutritional balance. Making sure that you are eating the right foods to keep your blood pressure at a healthy performing rate is the aim of this diet.

There are two levels of the DASH diet that you can partake in that are dependent in the sodium levels. If you wish to partake in the **Standard DASH Diet**, you will need to reduce your sodium intake to about 2,300 milligrams a day. If you wish to go BIG, then you can do the **Lower Sodium DASH Diet**, which is limited to about 1,500 milligrams of sodium a day. The lower sodium level is recommended for individuals that are 51 and older, African American, diabetic or have high blood pressure.

Chapter 2 – Recipes

Most dieters are burdened with the belief that they must eat less to lose more. This delusion is far from the truth. It's actually quite the opposite. Conversely, eating more can help you lose weight more efficiently. However, the trick is to eat the right foods, and making sure you eat enough of the right foods. Indulging in foods hold little to no nutritional value will not facilitate a healthy weight loss, no matter how small the amount. Foods that have been processed, refined, or genetically modified should never be included in anyone's diet. If you have these foods in your home, they should be alleviated from your diet immediately.

These foods have no significant nutrition, they cause a vast number of health issues, and offer no long-term or short-term benefits. Our bodies demand only the best. So, we need to meet those demands by only consuming organically-grown produce, grass-fed ruminants and dairy, free-range poultry, and wild-caught fish.

The nutritional value found in these foods is everything that our bodies need to lose weight and maintain health. This is what DASH Diet is centered around; wholesome nutrition and good eats! The recipes included in this book have been carefully selected to inspire you to eat good to look good.

Breakfast

Strawberry French Toast

Yield: Eight Servings
Active Time: 15 minutes
Cooking Time: 30 minutes
Total Time: 45 minutes

Ingredients
8 slices French bread
¾ cup apricot preserves (divided)
2 large egg whites
1 large egg, lightly beaten
½ cup fat-free cream cheese
¾ cup fat-free milk
⅛ tsp apple pie spice
½ tsp vanilla extract
Nonstick cooking spray

Cooking Directions
1. Preheat griddle to medium heat and lightly coat the griddle with cooking spray.
2. Combine cream cheese, and ¼ cup apricot preserves in a small bowl. Using a jagged knife, form a horizontal slit in each slice of bread. It should be a pocket that is halfway between the top and bottom of the bread crust. Add one tablespoon of the cheese mixture to each bread pocket. Set to the side.
3. Mix together milk, vanilla, apple spice, egg whites, and eggs in a small bowl. Dip both sides of each stuffed bread slice into the egg mixture.
4. Place each bread slice onto the preheated griddle, and cook for a minimum of 3 minutes or until lightly browned. Flip over after about one and a half minutes cooking.

5. In the meantime, melt the remaining apricot preserves in a small saucepan. Serve with the French toast.

Sausage and Potatoes Skillet

Yield: Six Servings
Active Time: 10 minutes
Cooking Time: 22 minutes
Total Time: 32 minutes

Ingredients
½ pound smoked turkey sausage, cooked and cut diagonally into ¼" slices
1 pound red potatoes, cut into ½" cubes
1 large onion, finely chopped
1 large green bell pepper, finely chopped
2 tbsp fresh thyme, finely chopped
2 tsp cumin seed, partially crushed
¼ tsp Himalayan Pink salt
¼ tsp freshly ground black pepper
4 tbsp unrefined extra-virgin olive oil

Cooking Directions
1. In a large skillet, heat 3 tablespoons olive oil over medium-high heat. Tilt skillet to evenly distribute oil. Add potatoes, bell pepper, and onion, and sauté for 10 to 12 minutes or until the potatoes are slightly tender. Stir occasionally.
2. Add the sausage and remaining olive oil to the potato mixture and cook for an additional 10 minutes, or until the potatoes are lightly browned. Stir frequently.
3. During the last minute of cooking, stir in cumin, thyme, salt, and pepper. Serve immediately.

Pineapple Omelet

Yield: Two Servings
Active Time: 10 minutes
Cooking Time: 10 minutes
Total Time: 20 minutes

Ingredients

6 large free-range eggs, lightly beaten
4 ounces shaved pastrami, chopped
2 garlic cloves, minced
1 cup fresh pineapple, chunked
4 ounces cremini mushrooms, roughly chopped
½ cup leek, finely chopped
½ cup feta cheese, crumbled
1 tsp cayenne pepper
Himalayan Pink salt, to taste
Freshly ground black pepper, to taste
Unrefined extra-virgin olive oil

Cooking Directions

1. In a large skillet, heat olive oil over medium-high heat. Toss in leeks, garlic, mushrooms, and pastrami. Sauté for a minimum of 5 minutes or until the vegetables are tender and pastrami is lightly browned.
2. Reduce heat. Add eggs, pineapple, cayenne, salt, and pepper. Allow the eggs to cook for about 3 to 5 minutes. Flip the omelet over and cook for an additional 3 to 5 minutes. Remove the omelet from the stove and add feta cheese to the eggs.
3. Flip the omelet close and cut in half. Serve immediately.

Rich and Crispy Millet Cakes

Yield: Six Servings
Active Time: 10 minutes
Cooking Time: 1 hour, 15 minutes
Total Time: 1 hour, 25 minutes

Ingredients
 1 cup millet
 ⅓ cup carrot, peeled and coarsely shredded
 ⅓ cup zucchini, peeled and coarsely shredded
 ¼ cup onion, finely chopped
 1 garlic cloves, minced
 ⅓ cup Parmesan cheese, grated
 1 ½ fresh thyme, finely choppe
 1 tsp lemon zest, freshly grated
 3 ½ water
 1 tbsp unrefined extra-virgin olive oil
 1 tsp cayenne pepper
 ¼ tsp freshly ground black pepper
 ½ Himalayan Pink salt

Cooking Directions
 1. In a large pot, heat the one tablespoon of olive oil over medium heat. Slowly stir in onion and sauté for about 2 to 5 minutes before stirring in garlic and millet. Cook for an additional 30 seconds, and pour in the water. Decrease the heat to low, stir in salt and cover to cook for about 20 minutes.
 2. Mix in Parmesan, carrot, zucchini, thyme, lemon zest, cayenne pepper, and black pepper. Bring the millet mixture to a simmer, and cook for uncovered for an additional 10 minutes or until the mixture has become soft

and thick. Remove from heat and set to the side to cool for about 10 minutes, covered.

3. With dampened hands, form the millet mixture into 12 patties. Patties should be about 3" in diameter.
4. Heat olive oil in a large skillet over medium heat. Add about 4 patties to the hot oil and cook on both sides for 3 to 5 minutes or until each patty is golden brown.
5. Repeat for the remaining batches.

Salmon and Herbs Stuffed Tomatoes

Yield: Four Servings
Active Time: 20 minutes
Cooking Time: 8 minutes
Total Time: 28 minutes

Ingredients
- 4 medium tomatoes, halved and seeds removed
- 8 ounces smoked Salmon, coarsely chopped
- 4 tbsp low-fat cream cheese
- 4 tbsp goat cheese, crumbled
- 2 tsp Parmesan cheese, grated
- 10 free-range eggs, lightly beaten
- 2 tbsp low-fat heavy cream
- ¼ cup fresh chives, finely chopped
- ½ tbsp fresh rosemary, finely chopped
- ½ tbsp fresh summer savory, finely chopped
- 1 tbsp fresh parsley, finely chopped

Cooking Directions
1. Set oven to broil, and line a large baking sheet with aluminum foil. Arrange tomato halves onto the prepared baking sheet. Set to the side.
2. In a medium bowl, combine rosemary, summer savory, and parsley. Mix well until the ingredients are blended. Set to the side.
3. Add olive oil to each tomato half and sprinkle with the herb mixture. Place into the oven to broil for a minimum of 3 minutes. Immediately turn off the broiler, and leave the tomatoes in the oven to roast as the oven cools off.

4. In a large skillet, heat olive oil over medium heat. Add eggs, heavy cream, smoked salmon, cream cheese, goat cheese, and chives. Using a fork, scramble the egg mixture for about 5 minutes or until the eggs are set.
5. Remove the tomatoes from the oven and stuff each with about ¼ of the egg mixture. Top each stuffed tomato with Parmesan cheese. Serve immediately.

Lunch

Yield: Six Servings
Active Time: 10 minutes
Marinating Time: 8 hours
Cooking Time: 10 minutes
Total Time: 8 hours, 20 minutes

Ingredients

2 pounds boneless, skinless, chicken beats, cut into 1" thick chunks
1 medium white onion
3 cups kale
4 garlic cloves, minced
2 green chile, seeded and chopped
1 jalapeño pepper, seeded and chopped
1 tbsp ginger root, freshly grated
2 tbsp lemon juice, freshly squeezed
1 tbsp lemon zest
¾ cup coconut water
¾ cup organic cashew butter (divided)
2 tbsp fresh cilantro, finely chopped
1 tsp garam masala
1 ½ tsp turmeric (divided)
⅔ cup unrefined extra-virgin olive oil (divided)
1 tsp Himalayan Pink salt
1 tsp freshly ground black pepper

Cooking Directions

1. In a large skillet, heat 3 tablespoon olive oil over medium heat. Toss in the jalapeño, green chile pepper, garlic, onion, and ginger. Sauté for a minimum of 2 to 3 minutes, and stir in kale. Cook for an additional 5 minutes or until

the kale leaves have wilted and the vegetables are tender. Remove from heat and set to the side to cool for about 5 minutes

2. Once the vegetable mixture is cooled, put the sautéed vegetables into a food processor. Add cilantro, lemon juice, lemon zest, ¼ cup cashew butter, ½ cup coconut water, garam masala, 1 teaspoon turmeric, salt, and pepper. Blend until the ingredients are pureed. Reserve about ¼ cup of the puree and set in the fridge to chill.

3. Place the chicken into a large bowl and pour the puree over the chicken. Rub the puree all over the chicken, and cover the bowl with plastic wrap. Allow the chicken to marinate for about 8 hours or overnight.

4. When chicken is ready to be cooked, set oven to 350 degrees.

5. Remove the chicken from the bowl, and skew an even amount of chicken onto wooden skewers.

6. Lightly grease a large baking sheet with olive oil, and add the chicken skewers to the baking sheet. Place in the oven to bake for about 15 to 20 minutes or until the juices of the chicken run clear.

7. In a medium bowl, combine the reserve puree, remaining turmeric, and remaining coconut water. Mix well to combine.

Cheesy Chicken Supreme Calzones

Yield: Six Servings
Active Time: 20 Minutes
Cooking Time: 15 minutes
Total Time: 35 minutes

Ingredients

12 ounces skinless, boneless chicken breasts, cooked and chopped/shredded
10 ounce refrigerated pizza dough
¼ cup celery, chopped
2 large Roma tomatoes, thinly sliced
¼ cup black olives, chopped
½ cup green bell peppers, chopped
½ cup red onion, thinly sliced
½ cup cremini mushrooms, thinly sliced
1 large free-range egg, lightly beaten
¾ cup Monterey Jack cheese, shredded
¾ cup Parmesan cheese
1 tbsp water
¾ cup tomato sauce
⅓ cup chives and onion cream cheese
2 tbsp fresh oregano, finely chopped
2 tbsp fresh basil, finely chopped
¼ tsp garlic powder
¼ tsp freshly ground black pepper
Unrefined extra-virgin olive oil

Cooking Directions

1. Set the oven to 425 degrees, and lightly grease a large baking sheet. Set to the side.
2. In a large bowl, combine chicken, cream cheese, mushrooms, Monterey Jack cheese, olives, celery, bell peppers, red onion, basil, oregano, garlic powder, and pepper. Mix well to combine and set to the side.

3. On a floured surface, unroll the pizza dough and cut into six 15"x10" rectangles. Add about one ounce tomato sauce and a few slices of Roma tomatoes to each.
4. Add even portion of the chicken mixture to each dressed rectangle. Brush all of the edges with water. Lift one of the outer edges and stretch dough over to the opposite edge. Seal the edges with a fork.
5. In a small bowl, mix together egg, ½ tablespoon olive oil, and ½ tablespoon water. Mix well until the mixture is emulsified.
6. Neatly arrange each calzone onto the prepared baking sheet. Brush the tops with egg mixture, and sprinkle about 1 ounce of parmesan cheese.
7. Place in the oven to bake for about 10 to 12 minutes. Remove from the oven immediately.

Oven-Fried Haddock & Chips

Yield: Four Servings
Active Time: 10 minutes
Cooking Time: 55 minutes
Total Time: 1 hour, 5 minutes

Ingredients

1 pound Haddock, cut into 4 even sections
1 ½ pound russet potatoes, cleaned, rinsed, and cut into ¼" thick wedges
¼ cup all-purpose flour
2 cups cornflakes
2 large egg whites, lightly beaten
1 ½ tsp Cajun seasoning (divided)
2 tsp dried parsley
¼ tsp Himalayan Pink salt
4 tsp unrefined extra-virgin olive oil
Olive Oil Cooking spray

Cooking Directions

1. Set oven to 425 degrees, and lightly grease a large baking sheet with olive oil. Add a wire rack onto another large baking sheet, and coat the wire rack with olive oil. Set to the side.
2. In a large bowl, combine potatoes, olive oil, ¾ teaspoon Cajun seasoning, and parsley. Mix well until all of the potato wedges are completely covered in oil mixture. Spread the coated potatoes in a single layer onto the prepared baking sheet (no rack). Place the potatoes in the oven to bake for a minimum of 30 to 35 minutes on the lower rack of the oven. Turn potatoes over every 10 minutes.
3. In the meantime, add cornflakes to a food processor and grind them into a coarse

mixture. Pour the crushed cornflakes into a shallow dish

4. Add egg whites to a separate shallow dish, and flour, salt, and remaining Cajun seasoning in another dish. Mix well to combine.
5. Batter each piece of Haddock in this order: add each piece of fish to the flour mixture, the egg white mixture, and the cornflake mixture. Be sure that all sides are well-coated. Place onto the prepared wire rack, and coat each side of the fish with the olive oil cooking spray.
6. Place the fish in the oven to back on the top rack for a minimum of 20 minutes or until the fish is crispy and golden brown.
7. Serve and enjoy immediately.

Stuffed Poblano Peppers

Yield: Two Servings
Active Time: 15 minutes
Cooking Time: 25 minutes
Total Time: 40 minutes

Ingredients
   2 Poblano peppers, stemmed
   4 large eggs, cracked and lightly chopped
   2 ramps, finely chopped
   1 large tomato, peeled and finely chopped
   2 cremini mushrooms, cleaned, rinsed, and chopped
   ½ cup goat cheese, crumbled
   2 tsp unrefined extra-virgin coconut oil, melted
   2 tbsp fresh cilantro, finely chopped
   2 tbsp fresh lemongrass, finely chopped
   Freshly ground black pepper, to taste
   Unrefined virgin olive oil

Cooking Directions
1. Set oven to 450 degrees, and lightly grease a large baking dish with olive oil.
2. Slit open Poblano peppers down one side, and remove the seeds. Lightly coat the peppers with olive oil, and place them in the baking dish with the cut side up. Open the peppers up, and place in the oven for a minimum of 20 to 30 minutes or until the skin is browned and the pepper becomes tender.
3. In the meantime, heat olive oil in a large skillet over medium-high heat. Beat together eggs, cilantro, and lemongrass. Gently fold in

mushrooms, tomatoes, ramps, and pepper. Pour mushroom mixture into the heated skillet. Scramble egg mixture to desired degree of doneness or for a minimum of 5 minutes.

4. When peppers are ready, spoon an even portion of the scrambled eggs into each pepper, and top each with goat cheese.
5. Place in the oven to bake for a minimum of 5 minutes or until the goat cheese is melted.

Yield: Four Servings
Active Time: 20 minutes
Cooking Time: 20 minutes
Total Time: 40 minutes

Ingredients

4 Mahi-Mahi fillets, skin removed
1 large grapefruit, peeled and chopped
2 tbsp lime juice, freshly squeezed
2 tsp organic raw honey
2 scallions, trimmed and thinly sliced
2 bunches watercress, thick stems removed
2 tbsp fresh parsley, finely chopped
2 tbsp fresh basil, finely chopped
1 avocado, peeled, cored, and cut into chunks
Unrefined virgin olive oil
Freshly ground black pepper

Cooking Directions

1. Lightly grease and preheat grill to medium-high heat, and place fish onto prepared grill.
2. Grill fish until the fish is easily flaked or for about 5 minutes on each side. Remove from heat, season with salt and pepper, and set to the side.
3. In a small bowl, mix together 3 tablespoons olive oil, lime juice, honey, scallions, parsley, basil, and pepper. Set to the side.
4. Ration watercress, avocado, and grapefruit evenly for each serving. Place fish on top of each of the watercress servings and drizzle with lime sauce.

Dinner

Slow-Cooker Mediterranean Venison

Yield: Five Servings
Active Time: 15 minutes
Cooking Time: 8 hours
Total Time: 8 hours, 15 minutes

Ingredients

2 pounds venison, cut into 1" thick cubes
¾ cup dried mangos, roughly chopped
¾ cup dates, roughly chopped
1 large yellow onion, thinly sliced
3 garlic cloves, minced
2 cups vegetable stock
1 cinnamon stick
1 ½ tsp ground ginger
1 tsp harissa
1 tsp saffron
2 tbsp fresh parsley, finely chopped
2 tbsp fresh cilantro, finely chopped
Unrefined extra-virgin olive oil

Cooking Directions

1. In a large bowl, combine cilantro, parsley, ginger, and venison. Toss and mix well to coat the meat. Set to the side.
2. At medium–high heat, add 1 tablespoon olive oil to a 2-quart crockpot. Place meat into the heated crock pot and sear venison on each side. Reduce the heat to low.
3. Heat 1 tablespoon olive oil over medium heat. Slowly stir in onions and garlic and sauté for a minimum of 5 minutes or until they become tender. Mix in vegetable stock and bring to a

boil. Immediately remove from the heat and pour into the crock pot along with the cinnamon stick.

4. Cook the mixture for about 5 hours and stir in dates, mango, and harissa. Cook for an additional 2 to 3 hours. Serve immediately.

Slow-Cooker Turkey Kielbasa and Sauerkraut

Yield: Four Servings
Active Time: 5 minutes
Cooking Time: 4 hours
Total Time: 4 hours, 5 minutes

Ingredients

- 1 ½ pound turkey kielbasa, chopped
- 1 large green apple, peeled, cored, and chopped
- ¾ cups sauerkraut
- 1 large yellow onion, finely chopped
- 2 tablespoons Dijon mustard
- 1 cup coconut water

Cooking Directions

1. Add all of the ingredients into a 2-quart slow cooker. Cook on high for about 4 hours.
2. Serve immediately.

Jerk Veggie Stir-Fry

Yield: Four Servings
Active Time: 10 minutes
Cooking Time: 20 minutes
Total Time: 30 minutes

Ingredients

- 2 large carrots, peeled and sliced
- 1 medium sweet onion, thinly sliced
- 1 cup broccoli, cut into florets
- 2 celery stalks, thinly sliced
- ½ cup water chestnuts, minced
- 1 cup fresh cremini mushrooms, thinly sliced
- 1 jalapeno, thinly sliced
- 1 medium red bell pepper, thinly sliced
- 1 medium yellow bell pepper, thinly sliced
- ¾ cups full-fat coconut milk
- 2 tbsp lime juice, freshly squeezed
- 3 tbsp unrefined extra-virgin coconut oil
- 1 ½ tbsp jerk seasoning
- Himalayan Pink salt, to taste
- Freshly ground black pepper, to taste

Cooking Directions

1. In a large wok, heat coconut oil over medium heat. Toss in onions to sauté for a minimum of 5 minutes or until the onions are transparent.
2. Stir in remaining vegetables and cook for about 10 minutes or until the vegetables are tender.
3. Slowly stir in coconut milk, lime juice, jerk seasoning, salt, and pepper. Cook for an additional 5 minutes or until the liquid has been

absorbed by the vegetables. Serve immediately.

Gouda Chicken Casserole

Yield: Six Servings
Active Time: 15 minutes
Cooking Time: 25 minutes
Total Time: 40 minutes

Ingredients
   8 boneless chicken thighs
   4 large avocado, peeled, cored, and thinly sliced
   1 large green bell pepper, sliced
   1 large cup green onions, thinly sliced
   4 garlic clove, minced
   ¾ cup heavy cream
   2 cups smoked Gouda cheese, shredded
   4 ounces low-fat cream cheese
   4 ounces low-fat sour cream
   4 tbsp lemon juice, freshly squeezed
   1 tbsp hot pepper sauce
   Himalayan Pink salt, to taste
   Freshly ground black pepper, to taste
   Unrefined extra-virgin olive oil

Cooking Directions
   1. Set oven to 350 degrees, and lightly grease a 9"x13" baking dish with olive oil.
   2. In a single layer, place the sliced avocados in the bottom of the prepared baking dish. Pour lemon juice over the avocados to prevent them from browning.
   3. In a large skillet, heat 2 tablespoons olive oil over medium-high heat. Add chicken thighs to the skillet, skin-side down. Cook each chicken

thigh for a minimum of 7 minutes on each side or until the juices run clear.

4. Add the chicken thighs to a large bowl, and flake using two forks. Stir in cheeses, bell pepper, onions, heavy cream, and sour cream.
5. Pour the chicken mixture over the avocados, and place in the oven to bake for about 20 to 25 minutes or until the casserole is golden brown and cheese bubbly.
6. Serve immediately.

Yield: Four Servings
Active Time: 20 minutes
Cooking Time: 10 minutes
Marinating Time: 8 hours or Overnight
Total Time: 8 hours, 30 minutes

Ingredients
½ pound boneless skinless chicken breasts, cut into 1" cubes
1 medium onion, finely chopped
¼ cup cashew butter
¼ cup sunflower seed butter
1 ½ tbsp organic apple cider vinegar
2 ¼ tsp lime juice, freshly squeezed
¾ tsp ground coriander
½ tsp ground cumin
½ garlic clove, minced
Himalayan Pink salt, to taste
Freshly ground black pepper, to taste
Unrefined extra-virgin olive oil

Cooking Directions
1. Combine sunflower seed butter, cashew butter, vinegar, lime juice, coriander, cumin, salt, pepper, cayenne pepper, and garlic in a small bowl. Stir until ingredients are well blended.
2. Add about 5 tablespoons of the sunflower seed/cashew butter mixture in a small container. Cover with a lid and place in the fridge to chill until ready to use.

3. Pour remaining mixture into to a large re-sealable plastic bag. Add onion and chicken cubes. Seal the bag.
4. Rotate or gently shake the bag to evenly coat the chicken. Place bag of chicken in a large bowl, and place in fridge. Allow to chill overnight.
5. The following day, remove the chicken from fridge. Drain the chicken and discard the marinade.
6. Preheat grill or broiler.
7. Divide the chicken cubes evenly, and thread onto four metal or soaked wooden skewers.
8. Lightly grease grill-rack with olive oil. Grill chicken kabobs over medium heat or broil the chicken at least 4" from the heat. Allow to cook for 4 to 5 minutes on each side or until the chicken is fully cooked. Remove chicken kabobs from the grill and brush with remaining marinade before serving.

Dessert

Homemade Nutty Chocolatey Coconut Ice Cream

Yield: One Serving
Active Time: 15 minutes
Cooking Time: 4 hours
Total Time: 4 hours, 15 minutes

Ingredients
1 can full-fat heavy cream milk
1 tbsp cashew butter
1 tbsp almond butter
4 egg yolks
¼ cup cacao nibs
3 tbsp organic raw honey
¼ cup silvered almonds, finely chopped
4 tbsp vanilla extract

Cooking Directions
1. Bring water to a boil in a double broiler.
2. Pour coconut milk, almond butter, cashew butter, cacao nibs, and vanilla extract. Stirring constantly, heat the coconut milk mixture enough to melt the chocolate. *(***Be sure not to allow the mixture to boil.)*
3. In a separate bowl, whisk together the egg yolks. Whisking vigorously, add about ¼ cup of the coconut milk mixture to the egg yolks.
4. Pour the tempered egg yolks into the coconut mixture, and beat until it forms into custard. *(***Be sure not to cook the eggs and the double broiler is not too hot!)*
5. Pour the custard into a large bowl and allow it to cool at room temperature.

6. Once the custard reaches the room temperature, and add to an ice cream maker and freeze (be sure to follow the manufacturer's directions).
7. Enjoy at your desired degree of softness.

S'Mores Pie

Yield: Eight Servings
Active Time: 15 minutes
Cooking Time: 2 hours
Total Time: 10 hours, 15 minutes

Ingredients
- 1 (9") graham cracker pie crust
- 4 ounces unsweetened chocolate, chopped
- 1 cup brown sugar (divided)
- 4 egg whites
- ¼ tsp cream of tartar
- ⅓ fat-free half-and-half
- 2 tsp vanilla extract (divided)

Cooking Directions
1. Set oven to 225 degrees.
2. In a medium saucepan, cook half-and-half and ½ cup brown sugar over medium heat. Stir constantly. When sugar is fully dissolved, add 1 tsp vanilla and chocolate. Simmer and stir until chocolate melts. Remove from heat and pour chocolate mixture into the graham cracker pie crust. Set aside.
3. In a large bowl, beat together egg whites, cream of tartar, and remaining vanilla extract using an electric mixer. Beat until the egg white mixture stiff peaks, while slowly stirring in remaining brown sugar (1 tbsp at a time). Allow brown sugar to dissolve. Spread egg white mixture evenly over the chocolate filling.
4. Place in the oven to bake for a minimum of 2 hours, and turn oven off and let the pie sit in oven overnight or for 8 hours.

Cara and Mel's Bread Pudding

Yield: Ten Servings
Active Time: 15 minutes
Cooking Time: 45 minutes
Total Time: 120 minutes

Ingredients
   12 slices wheat bread
   1 large green apple, sliced
   ¼ cup pecans
   1 ½ cup low-fat milk
   6 eggs beaten, lightly beaten
   ½ cup low-fat butter
   1 cup brown sugar
   2 tbsp light corn syrup
   1 tsp vanilla extract
   ½ tsp almond extract
   Cooking spray

Cooking Directions
1. In a medium saucepan, heat butter, corn syrup, and sugar over medium heat. Simmer for about 5 minutes or until mixture thickens. Remove from heat and pour into prepared baking dish and sprinkle with pecans. Place apple sliced over the pecans, and top with 2 layers of bread slices.
2. In a large bowl, whisk together eggs, milk, vanilla extract, almond extract, and salt. Pour mixture over the bread and caramel mixture. Cover and refrigerate for 60 minutes.
3. Preheat oven to 350 degrees.
4. Remove casserole from fridge and bake for 40 to 45 minutes or until the casserole is golden brown. Serve hot.

Lemon-Lime Bars

Yield: Thirty-Six Bars
Active Time: 25 minutes
Cooking Time: 35 minutes
Total Time: 3 hours, 30 minutes

Ingredients
Crust:
- 4 cups all-purpose flour
- ½ cup arrowroot starch
- ½ tsp baking soda
- ½ cup organic raw honey
- 2 tsp vanilla extract
- 1 cup unrefined extra-virgin coconut oil
- ½ tsp Himalayan Pink salt

Topping:
- 4 large eggs, lightly beaten
- ¾ cup organic raw honey
- ¼ cup lemon juice, freshly squeezed
- ¼ cup lime juice, freshly squeezed
- 5 tbsp arrowroot starch

Cooking Directions
1. Set oven to 325 degrees and lightly grease a 9"x13" with coconut oil.
2. Combine flour, starch, salt, and baking soda in a large bowl. Mix well to combine the ingredients, and form a well in the center.
3. In a separate bowl, mix together honey, vanilla extract, and coconut oil. Using a fork, bet the ingredients together until the ingredients are emulsified. Pour into the well of the dry ingredients.

4. Mix well to combine and pour into the prepared baking dish. Press down to the batter into the baking dish.
5. Place in the oven to bake for a minimum of 30 minutes or until the crust becomes golden brown. Remove the crust from the oven and set to the side to cool for about 15 minutes.
6. In the meantime, combine all of the topping ingredients in a large bowl. Using a whisk or fork, mix the ingredients together until a smooth consistency is reached. Spread over the crust.
7. Place in the oven to bake for an additional 20 minutes.

Yield: 8 Slices
Active Time: 10 minutes
Cooking Time: 0 minutes
Chill Time: 2 hours
Total Time: 2 hours, 10 minutes

Ingredients
Filing:

- 4 avocados, peeled, cored, and diced
- 8 ounces cream cheese
- 8 tbsp organic raw honey
- 1 cup unrefined extra-virgin coconut oil
- ⅔ cup lime juice, freshly squeezed

Crust:

- ½ cup Medjool dates, roughly chopped
- ¼ cup unsweetened coconut, shredded
- 1 ½ cup almond flour
- ¼ coconut flour
- 1 tbsp almond butter
- 2 tbsp organic raw honey

Cooking Directions
Crust:

1. Lightly grease a 9" springform pan with coconut oil.
2. Add dates, shredded coconut, flour, and honey to a food processor. Pulse until the mixture becomes crumbly. Dump the mixture into the prepared springform pan and press to form a crust.

Filing:

3. Blend together avocados, cream cheese, honey, coconut oil, and lime juice into food processor until the mixture becomes smooth. Pour into the crust and smooth out the top.
4. Place in the fridge to chill for about 2 hours.

Snack

Yield: One Serving
Active Time: 5 minutes
Blending Time: 2 to 3 minutes
Total Time: 7 to 8 minutes

Ingredients

- 1 large egg
- 1 large avocado, peeled, cored, and chopped
- 1 large frozen banana, chopped (peel before freezing)
- 2 tbsp ground flax seeds
- 4 tbsp organic raw red walnut butter
- 2 tbsp cacao nibs
- 2 ounces low-fat cream cheese
- ½ cup low-fat heavy cream
- ½ cup organic coconut milk
- 1 tbsp unrefined extra-virgin coconut oil
- 5 drops Stevia
- 1 vanilla bean

Directions

1. Add all of the ingredients to the blender, and puree until all of the ingredients become completely smooth.
2. Pour into your favorite glass and enjoy!

Mini Strawberry Rhubarb Lattice Pies

Yield: Six Mini-Lattice pies
Active Time: 45 minutes
Bake Time: 30 minutes
Total Time: 1 hour, 15 minutes

Ingredients
- 3 cups fresh rhubarb, chopped
- 3 cups fresh strawberries
- ¼ cup turbinado sugar
- 1 ½ cups 100% pure cane sugar, granulated
- ½ cup cornstarch
- 1 box refrigerated pie crusts, softened
- 1 egg white, beaten
- 1 tbsp butter
- 2 tbsp lime juice
- Ground ginger to taste
- Ground cinnamon to taste
- Cooking spray

Cooking Directions
1. Set oven to 375 degrees, and coat a 24 cup muffin pan with cooking spray. Set aside.
2. Melt butter in a large skillet over medium-high heat, and add rhubarb. Sauté rhubarb for about 7 minutes or until rhubarb becomes soft. Mix in strawberries and granulated sugar and cook until the mixture becomes thick. Immediately remove from heat and stir in lime juice, ginger, and cinnamon. Add rhubarb/strawberry mixture and cornstarch to blender and puree.
3. Unroll pie crusts, and cut three rounds from each crust and press into all muffin cups.

Have the crusts hanging over the sides of the muffin cups. Trim crusts.

4. Fill each crust-lined muffin cup with at least ½ cup rhubarb/strawberry mixture.

5. Thinly slice the remaining pie crusts into 42 strips that are about 3" long. Weave 8 strips together to create lattice square. Cut square with 2 ½" round cutter. Place lattice round over top of filling in crust-lined muffin cup. Roll hanging pie crust edge to meet lattice top. Brush each mini pie with butter, and top with turbinado sugar.

6. Bake until the filling begins to set and crust is golden brown or for a minimum 25 to 30 minutes.

Mini Caesar Salads

Yield: Sixteen Mini-Muffins
Active Time: 15 minutes
Bake Time: 10 minutes
Total Time: 25 minutes

Ingredients

8 - 8" flour tortillas
2 boneless, skinless, grilled chicken breasts, shredded
3 tbsp Caesar dressing
½ cup romaine lettuce, finely chopped
¼ cup whole kernel corn, cooked
⅜ cup Parmesan cheese, grated (divided)
4 grape tomatoes, quartered
Cooking spray

Cooking Directions

1. Set oven to 375 degrees, and coat a 16 cup mini muffin pan with cooking spray. Sprinkle about 2 tbsp Parmesan cheese onto the sides and bottoms of each prepared cups. Set aside.
2. Cut out 16 (2 ½") rounds from tortillas, and place each round into each muffin cup to form a tortilla cup. Place into in oven and allow to bake for a minimum of 5 minutes. Remove from oven and allow to cool.
3. In a medium bowl, stir together chicken and Caesar dressing. Set aside.
4. Add an even portion of lettuce to each tortilla cup. Top each cup of lettuce with chicken coated with dressing. Sprinkle with remaining cheese, corn, and tomatoes. Serve immediately.

Yield: Forty-Eight Servings
Active Time: 30 minutes
Bake Time: 15 minutes
Total Time: 50 minutes

Ingredients
½ cup low-fat cream cheese, softened
½ cup sour cream
1 tsp lemon-pepper seasoning
2 tbsp fresh chives, chopped
2 tsp small capers, drained
1 ¼ cup frozen corn, thawed
½ smoked salmon, flaked
2 (8 ounce) cans crescent dinner rolls, refrigerated
¼ tsp Himalayan Pink salt
Cooking spray

Cooking Directions
1. Set oven to 375 degrees and coat a 48 mini muffin pan or two 24 mini muffin pans with cooking spray. Set aside.
2. Combine cream cheese, sour cream, lemon-pepper seasoning, chives, capers, corn, and salt in a medium bowl, and stir until well blended. Gently fold in salmon.
3. Unroll crescent rolls and divide into 8 rectangles. Press down on perforations in the center to seal, and then cut the rectangles into six 2" squares. Place each square into each prepared mini muffin cup, and press against all sides of the cup. Add 1 tablespoon of the salmon filling into each pie square.

4. Bake for a minimum of 10 to 18 minutes or until the mini muffin is golden brown. Allow to cool for 2 minutes, and remove from pan.

Quinoa with Peaches and Creamy Yogurt

Yield: Two Servings
Active Time: 15 minutes
Cooking Time: 15 minutes
Total Time: 30 minutes

Ingredients

- ½ cup pre-rinsed quinoa
- 1 cup water
- ½ tsp ground cinnamon
- ½ tsp ground nutmeg
- ½ large fresh peach, pitted and chopped
- ¼ cup fat-free Greek yogurt
- 1 tbsp honey, or to taste
- ½ pinch ground nutmeg
- 1 ½ tsp lime juice, or to taste

Cooking Directions

1. In a medium saucepan, bring 2 cups of water to a boil. Once water begins to boil, stir in quinoa and reduce heat to low and allow to simmer for at least 15 to 20 minutes or until tender.
2. Remove from heat and drain excess water. Stir in cinnamon and 1 tsp of nutmeg.
3. In a medium bowl, combine yogurt and chopped peaches. Stir until peaches are well coated.
4. Serve quinoa in a serving bowl, and top each serving with about 2 tablespoons of the peach yogurt.
5. Pour a small portion of honey over the top and sprinkle with nutmeg.
6. Enjoy!

Spinach Triangles

Yield: Three Servings
Active Time: 15 minutes
Cooking Time: 40 minutes
Total Time: 55 minutes

Ingredients

    10 ounces fresh spinach, rinsed and stems
    removed
    ⅜ medium onions, finely chopped
    1 garlic clove, minced
    2 cups Monterey Jack cheese, shredded
    9 ounces whole-wheat flour
    ¼ cup warm water
    2 tbsp lemon juice, freshly squeezed
    1 ¼ tsp fresh basil leaves, finely chopped
    1 ¼ tsp fresh mint leaves, finely chopped
    ¼ tsp active dry yeast
    ¼ tsp 100% pure cane sugar
    ⅛ tsp garlic salt
    ¼ tsp Himalayan Pink salt
    1 ¼ tsp unrefined extra-virgin olive oil

Cooking Directions

1. Set oven to 450 degrees. (If you have a pizza stone, place the pizza stone in the oven while the oven heats up.)
2. Stir together sugar, yeast, and hot water in a small bowl and set aside. Allow bubbles to form in the yeast, and then pour in salt and olive oil.
3. In a large bowl, combine flour and yeast mixture to form into a partially, soft dough.
4. On a lightly floured surface, knead the dough with your hands using slightly heavy pressure. Continue kneading the dough until it reaches a

smooth and soft texture. This process should take at least 15 minutes.

5. Place dough in a large bowl, and cover bowl with a clean towel to allow dough to rise and rest.
6. Roughly chop spinach.
7. In a large pot, add salt, water and spinach. Bring this to a boil and allow to cook for 2 minutes, or until the spinach has wilted.
8. Drain the spinach well and return to the pot. Add cheese, onions, lemon juice, garlic, basil, mint, and garlic salt to the spinach. Allow to cook until the cheese has melted or for about 5 to 10 minutes.
9. Remove dough from bowl, and cut into golf-ball size pieces. Roll the pieces into 5-inch wide disks. Be sure the disks are about ¼ inch thick.
10. In the center of each "disk", dump 1 tablespoon of the spinach filing.
11. After all disks have been dressed with spinach filing, fold up three sides of the disk to form into a triangle. Be sure to leave a small hole in the center to allow steam to release while baking.
12. Bake for 10 to 15 minutes, or until golden brown.

Chapter 3 – Tips

Here are some helpful tips to supplement your DASH Diet. If you are participating in this diet to lose weight, you will find these tips to be very beneficial to the weight loss process.

Exercise

Physical exercise has a positive influence on weight loss. Physical activities will increase the speed at which you burn calories, and will also assist your thyroid in producing healthy hormones that will help your maintain and increase your metabolism.

Get Support

Making changes to your lifestyle and eating habits can be very difficult, but having someone there to support you makes it easier. Get with a close friend or family member and discuss what you know about DASH Diet and see if they would like to try the diet with you. If you are not able to find anyone that is interested, all hope is not lost. There are numerous DASH support groups on Facebook, social media websites. The Internet is filled with websites dedicated to DASH Eating. Become a part of one of the many DASH communities, and you will be able to participate in forum discussions and even ask for advice. You can even find some great DASH Diet apps on your phone.

No More Microwaving

The microwave oven is just one of those inventions that has destroyed the overall health of mankind. Microwaves are not meant for human consumption. However, each time you heat your food in the microwave, you are consuming microwaves. These dangerous machines not only contaminate your food with harmful radiation, it removes all of the nutritional value from your food. So, it is best to avoid the microwave to the best of your abilities.

Things to Remember

Even though the DASH diet has many benefits, there are some things that you should be aware of before you begin the diet. Let's take a look below.

- Even though this diet includes lean meats, it is vital to eat in moderation. Eating too much meat increases the risk of a colon and other forms of cancer. So, take it easy on the meat.

- This diet is not meant for you to reduce your food or calorie intake. This diet only requires you to switch your eating habits from unhealthy to healthy. So, eat as much as your body requires.

- This diet requires a great amount of cooking. If your schedule is very busy, it is recommended to prepare your meals ahead of time. This will save you a lot of time.

- Talk with your doctor before you begin the DASH Diet. The diet may possibly affect some pre-existing medical conditions.

Conclusion

Embarking on a new diet can be very intimidating and when you don't really know what to expect. However, there are certain things that you can do to enhance the flavors of your dishes such as using salt, healthy forms of fat or using fruits and vegetables to bring out the flavors of your dishes. Follow these tasty recipes to make the most delicious of your journey to a healthier you.

The DASH Diet will assist you in breaking your addiction to high-sugar, high-calorie foods by encouraging you to implement more fruits, vegetables, whole-grains, and lean protein into your diet. Everyone's diet lacks nutritional balance, with the DASH diet you will be able to obtain the balance you need. However, this requires some effort, and dedication. To achieve the best results and benefits from this diet, it is vital to eat the right foods and the correct amount of foods. If you really want achieve the ultimate results, it is recommended to check all food labels. There are a lot of hidden fats, sugars, and carbs out there just lurking in some your favorite for, just waiting to throw you off of your path to DASH Diet success.

By following this diet plan you'll be able to lose your desired amount of weight in your ideal amount of time. It's all about natural weight loss by controlling your food and calorie intake. This diet plan does not involve starving yourself. Remember you are losing weight to look good and be healthy, and not to look sick and malnourished. Always consult with your physician before proceeding with any diet plan. As long as you try your best to spice up your dish and remember to use as many fruits and veggies as possible, all of the dishes in this book will be easy to love.

Hopefully you have found at least one recipe that you love in this very carefully selected compilation. There are plenty of healthy choices of breakfast, lunch, dinner and dessert recipes here that you can make to impress your friends or family.

www.ingramcontent.com/pod-product-compliance
Lightning Source LLC
Chambersburg PA
CBHW070818290526
45795CB00002B/750